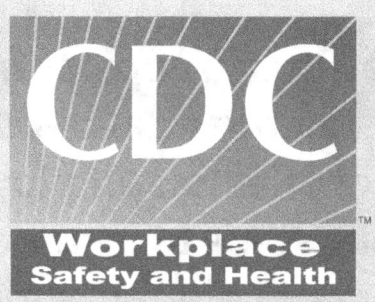

Chemotherapy Drug Evaluation at a Veterinary Teaching Hospital – Michigan

James Couch, CIH, MS, REHS/RS
John Gibbins, DVM, MPH
Thomas Connor, PhD

Health Hazard Evaluation Report
HETA 2010-0068-3156
April 2012
Revised April 2013

DEPARTMENT OF HEALTH AND HUMAN SERVICES
Centers for Disease Control and Prevention

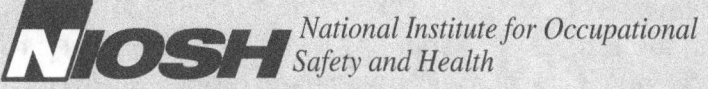 National Institute for Occupational Safety and Health

The employer shall post a copy of this report for a period of 30 calendar days at or near the workplace(s) of affected employees. The employer shall take steps to insure that the posted determinations are not altered, defaced, or covered by other material during such period. [37 FR 23640, November 7, 1972, as amended at 45 FR 2653, January 14, 1980].

Revision Summary: The original final report contained technical inaccuracies in the process description, erroneous references to the chemotherapeutic drug carmustine which was never used by the veterinary hospital, and mistakenly cited linear feet per minute measurements as cubic feet per minute measurements.

CONTENTS

ABBREVIATIONS

ACGIH®	American Conference of Governmental Industrial Hygienists
BSC	Biological safety cabinet
CDC	Centers for Disease Control and Prevention
CFR	Code of Federal Regulations
HEPA	High-efficiency particulate air
HHE	Health hazard evaluation
IARC	International Agency for Research on Cancer
IV	Intravenous
LOD	Limit of detection
LOQ	Limit of quantitation
NAICS	North American Industry Classification System
ND	Not detected
NIOSH	National Institute for Occupational Safety and Health
ng/sample	Nanograms per sample
ng/100 cm^2	Nanograms per 100 square centimeters
OEL	Occupational exposure limit
OSHA	Occupational Safety and Health Administration
PEL	Permissible exposure limit
PPE	Personal protective equipment
REL	Recommended exposure limit
STEL	Short-term exposure limit
TLV®	Threshold limit value
WEEL™	Workplace environmental exposure level

The National Institute for Occupational Safety and Health (NIOSH) received a confidential employee request for a health hazard evaluation from a veterinary teaching hospital in Michigan. Employees were concerned about reproductive problems and hair loss that they associated with work-related exposures to chemotherapy drugs.

What NIOSH Did

- We evaluated the facility on September 13–15, 2010.

- We took surface wipe and air samples for cyclophosphamide, ifosfamide, and doxorubicin. These substances are chemotherapy drugs.

- We talked with employees privately about their work.

- We discussed the occupational risks associated with chemotherapy drugs to the employer, employees, and students.

- We met with university officials in charge of the veterinary teaching hospital's occupational health and safety program.

What NIOSH Found

- Cyclophosphamide and ifosfamide were found in 4 of 44 surface wipe samples.

- Cyclophosphamide and ifosfamide were not found in air samples.

- Some employees reported headache, nausea, and abnormal menstruation. These symptoms have been reported with occupational exposure to chemotherapy drugs in earlier studies. They also have other causes.

- No employees reported hair loss at the time of our interviews.

- Most employees were not satisfied with the occupational health and safety program, particularly in the areas of training, supervisor communication, and re-use of disposable personal protective equipment.

- Employees did not report using personal protective equipment every time they administered chemotherapy drugs.

What Managers Can Do

- Ask employees to select training topics. They may also be able to assist in developing training materials.

- Tell employees about safe work practices involving chemotherapy drugs.

- Limit employee access to the pharmacy, chemotherapy drug preparation room, and administration area. Keep doors leading to these areas closed as much as possible.

- Use a biological safety cabinet that does not recirculate exhaust air when you prepare a volatile chemotherapy drug such as Mustargen®.

- Post "Chemotherapy Drug Administration in Progress" signs when preparing and administering chemotherapy drugs to remind staff to follow proper procedures.

- Wear two pairs of chemotherapy protective gloves when decontaminating the biological safety cabinet and when administering chemotherapy drugs. You should also wear a protective gown for these tasks.

- Use separate cleaning supplies for the chemotherapy drug preparation room and administration area. Store these supplies in the area where they are used.

- Follow the hospital's procedure when handling soiled bedding and blankets used by animals receiving chemotherapy.

- Place color-coded collars on animals recently treated with chemotherapy drugs. Treat their body fluids as chemotherapy drug spills.

- Do not allow eating and drinking in areas where chemotherapy drugs are handled, administered, or stored.

What Employees Can Do

- Follow standard operating procedures that have been established for work tasks. Always wear the required personal protective equipment.

- Attend health and safety training and participate in safety meetings.

- Do not eat or drink in areas where chemotherapy drugs are handled or stored.

Summary

NIOSH investigators evaluated chemotherapy drug exposures and their possible relationship to reproductive problems and hair loss among employees at a veterinary teaching hospital. Cyclophosphamide and ifosfamide were detected on some surface wipe samples, but not in the air. We could not determine if the health effects reported by employees were work related; however, similar effects have been reported with occupational exposure to chemotherapy drugs in other studies.

In February 2010, NIOSH received a confidential employee HHE request concerning exposure to chemotherapy drugs at a university veterinary teaching hospital (veterinary hospital) in Michigan. Employees were concerned that exposure to chemotherapy drugs may cause adverse health effects such as reproductive problems and hair loss.

We visited the veterinary hospital in September 2010 and observed work practices and workplace conditions. We talked with employees about their health and workplace concerns related to chemotherapy drugs. We collected surface wipe and air samples for the chemotherapy drugs cyclophosphamide, ifosfamide, and doxorubicin. We gave a presentation on the occupational risks associated with chemotherapy and other hazardous drugs to the employer, employees, and students. We also met with university officials responsible for the veterinary hospital's occupational health and safety program.

Cyclophosphamide was detected in 4 of 44 surface wipe samples, ranging from ND (< 5 ng/100 cm^2) to 240 ng/100 cm^2. All detectable levels of cyclophosphamide were found in the chemotherapy drug preparation room and administration area. Ifosfamide was detected in 2 of 44 surface wipe samples, ranging from ND (< 2 ng/100 cm^2) to 37 ng/100 cm^2. We detected neither cyclophosphamide nor ifosfamide in the air samples. Doxorubicin was not detected (LOD = 7 ng/sample) in any of the surface wipe or air samples, but we believe the recovery of doxorubicin from these samples may have been poor because of the length of time the samples were stored frozen before analysis.

Most employees we talked with were not satisfied with the health and safety program, particularly in the areas of training, supervisor communication, and required re-use of disposable PPE. A few employees reported that they did not always wear appropriate PPE when administering chemotherapy drugs. Three employees reported health effects (headache, nausea, and abnormal menstruation) that have been associated with chemotherapy exposure in prior studies, but that also have a variety of other etiologies. No employees reported hair loss at the time of our evaluation.

We were unable to determine if the health effects reported by employees were work related. However, similar effects have been reported with occupational exposure to chemotherapy drugs in other studies. We have provided recommendations that may reduce chemotherapy drug exposure, address employee concerns about their workplace health and safety program, and lead to more consistent work practices and personal protective equipment use.

Keywords: NAICS 541940 (Veterinary Services), chemotherapy, oncology, anti-neoplastic, hazardous drugs, veterinary, cyclophosphamide, ifosfamide, doxorubicin, surface wipe samples, air samples

On February 26, 2010, NIOSH received a confidential employee request for an HHE at a veterinary teaching hospital ("veterinary hospital") in Michigan. The veterinary hospital provides routine care and oncology services to large and small animals. Canines and felines constitute the majority of the oncology department's patients. Veterinary hospital employees were concerned about adverse health effects from the use of chemotherapy drugs in the oncology department.

On September 13-15, 2010, NIOSH investigators visited the veterinary hospital and met with representatives of the employer, two employee unions, and students. During the opening meeting we discussed surface and air sampling for chemotherapy drug exposures. We toured the veterinary hospital to observe work processes, practices, and workplace conditions. We collected surface wipe and air samples and analyzed them for cyclophosphamide, ifosfamide, and doxorubicin. We also interviewed staff confidentially to discuss their work practices, medical history, and symptoms as well as their personal assessment of training and supervision. We held a closing meeting on September 15, 2010, with employer and union representatives to summarize our activities and provide preliminary findings. We sent a letter dated October 13, 2010, with preliminary findings.

Process Description

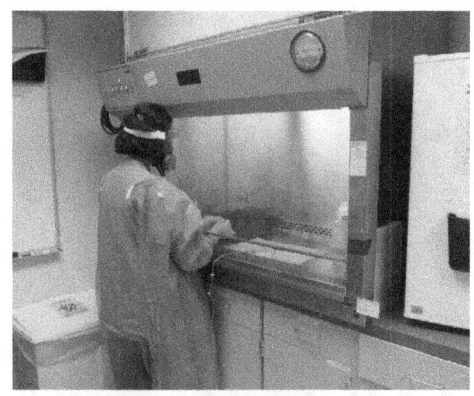

Figure 1. Veterinary technician wearing PPE while preparing chemotherapy drugs in a Class 2 BSC.

Chemotherapy drugs were received at the veterinary hospital pharmacy as powders, liquids, or premixed solutions. Pharmacy personnel dispensed oral drugs on a per patient basis for owner administration at home. Owners received instructions on how to safely handle these medications. Drugs that were administered at the veterinary hospital were transported to the chemotherapy drug preparation room (Room D157) where they were refrigerated and stored until needed. The drugs were removed and prepared in a Class 2 BSC in the chemotherapy preparation room. Air exhausted from the BSC passed through a HEPA filter and was recirculated back into the room (Figure 1).

Animals typically receive several diagnostic procedures before receiving chemotherapy drugs to ensure that they are healthy enough to receive the treatment. Animals were kenneled in the administration area (Room D159) until cleared for treatment. Once cleared, animals received the chemotherapy drugs in

INTRODUCTION (CONTINUED)

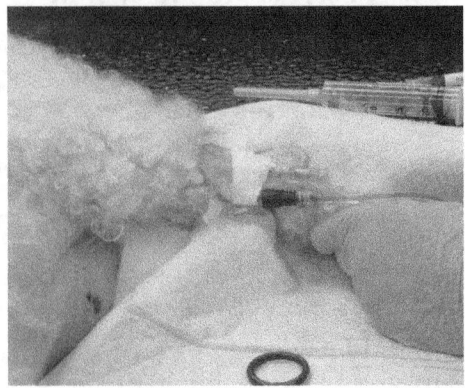

Figure 2. Intravenous administration procedure for doxorubicin.

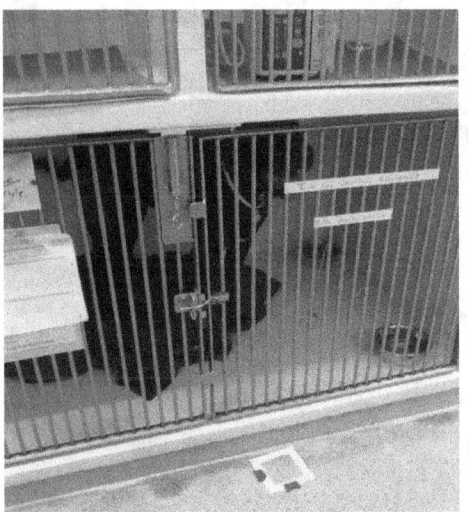

Figure 3. A chemotherapy drug-treated canine in a labeled kennel. The label warned employees of potential chemotherapy drug cross contamination and identified the chemotherapy drug used.

a procedure that required at least two employees or students to restrain the animals for IV catheter placement and drug administration. Animals were placed on the treatment table and prepared by shaving and disinfecting the area where the IV catheter was placed. The administering technician then injected the chemotherapy drug. Figure 2 illustrates a chemotherapy drug injection process.

After treatment, animals were removed from the table and kenneled in the administration area or in cages or runs in adjacent areas (Figure 3). Employees then decontaminated the treatment table and surrounding floor with a bleach solution. The IV tubing, bag, and other potentially contaminated items were placed in chemotherapy-approved disposal containers, and the area was wiped with a 10% bleach solution and allowed to dry.

After receiving chemotherapy, animals were occasionally taken to radiology/ultrasound, the nursing care unit, or the critical care unit for further diagnostics, medical care, or observation only on an as-needed basis. Animals also were walked indoors or outside the veterinary hospital. After completing treatment, animals were discharged to their owners with instructions on how to safely handle the animal's urine, feces, and vomit that could be contaminated with chemotherapy drugs. The owners were also told how to safely clean up accidents and were informed about PPE that could be worn when cleaning up after the animals.

On September 13–15, 2010, we collected surface wipe and air samples for cyclophosphamide, ifosfamide, and doxorubicin, chemotherapy drugs commonly used at this veterinary hospital. Appendix A contains additional sampling and analytical information. Surface wipe samples were collected in the chemotherapy drug preparation room and administration area. We collected samples on surfaces where we believed the potential for chemotherapy drug contamination was greatest. Offices, employee break rooms, and public reception areas where no PPE was used were also sampled to learn whether chemotherapy drugs were inadvertently spread beyond treatment areas.

We collected area air samples in the chemotherapy drug preparation room and administration area and a background area air sample from a clerical area. Because cyclophosphamide, ifosfamide, and doxorubicin have low vapor pressures (meaning that they are unlikely to volatilize during administration) we used an air flow sampling rate of 15 liters per minute to increase our ability to detect low airborne concentrations. We also visually examined the BSC, reviewed its certification records, and asked employees and managers about their work practices when using the BSC.

We held confidential interviews with 13 randomly selected employees who directly worked with chemotherapy drugs. Job titles included veterinarians and licensed veterinary and pharmacy technicians. We asked about their work history, health concerns, and medical history. We asked for their personal assessment of safety policies and procedures, knowledge about recommended disposal methods for chemotherapy drugs and supplies, and satisfaction with the veterinary hospital's health and safety program. We also asked about the PPE used when they handled chemotherapy drugs and their perceptions about communication with their supervisor about safety issues related to chemotherapy drug handling and administration.

We informally talked with employees and observed work practices in other areas of the veterinary hospital including radiology, critical care and nursing care units, other patient wards, the laundry, and grounds keeping. We assessed employees' knowledge about handling animals that had received chemotherapy drugs, disposal of chemotherapy drugs, and cleaning procedures.

Surface Wipe and Air Sampling

As shown in the table, most of the surface sample results (40 of 44) were below the LOD of 5 ng/sample for cyclophosphamide and 2 ng/sample for ifosfamide. The highest result, 240 ng/100 cm^2 for cyclophosphamide, was collected beneath the BSC grate, and all detectable levels of cyclophosphamide and ifosfamide were from samples collected in and around the BSC in the chemotherapy drug preparation room (D157). This suggests the potential for chemotherapy drug exposures to employees compounding or mixing in the BSC. No doxorubicin was detected (LOD = 7 ng/sample) in any of the surface wipe samples. However, the recovery of doxorubicin from these samples may have been poor because the samples were frozen prior to analysis.

Cyclophosphamide and ifosfamide were not detected (minimum detectable concentration was 0.07 nanograms per cubic meter for a 7,000-liter air sample) in general area air samples collected from the chemotherapy drug preparation room, the administration area, and an office behind admissions. Doxorubicin was not detected (minimum detectable concentration was 0.1 nanograms per cubic meter for a 7,000-liter air sample) but its recovery may have been poor because the samples were stored frozen prior to analysis.

Employee Interviews

The median age of the 13 employees we interviewed was 34 years (range: 27 to 55 years). The median number of years employees had worked with chemotherapy drugs, either at this veterinary hospital or in other workplaces, was 4.5 years with a range of less than 1 to 30 years. Most employees denied any health symptoms while handling or working around chemotherapy drugs. Three employees reported headache, and one reported occasional nausea and facial flushing. One employee reported abnormal menstruation that began after starting work with chemotherapy drugs. No employees reported hair loss at the time of the interviews.

When asked how satisfied they were with their work area's present health and safety program, 10 of 13 employees reported "not satisfied," while three employees reported being "somewhat satisfied" or "satisfied." When asked if written policies were available at their work area regarding PPE use, 11 of 13 reported no written policies were available. Regarding self-reported

RESULTS
(CONTINUED)

Table. Chemotherapy drugs in surface wipe samples collected on September 13–15, 2010

Location	Sample Description	Results, ng/100 cm²	
		Cyclophosphamide	Ifosfamide
Pharmacy	Receiving table	ND	ND
	Plastic bin for transporting chemotherapy drugs	ND	ND
	Desktop near oral chemotherapy pill cabinet	ND	ND
	Countertop adjacent to small refrigerator and BSC	ND	ND
	Top of chemotherapy waste disposal bin	ND	ND
Drug Preparation Room (D157)	Countertop adjacent to small refrigerator and BSC	ND	ND
	BSC working surface	77	ND
	BSC airfoil	ND	ND
	BSC top portion of cabinet (estimated area)	ND	ND
	BSC underneath the grate	240	37
	Floor directly in front of BSC	(5)	29
Administration Area (D159)	Chemotherapy drug administration table (stainless steel area)	ND	ND
	Tool cart with various supplies and instruments	ND	ND
	Exam table on the soft padding	ND	ND
	Exam table on the soft padding after doxorubicin administration	(11)	ND
	Floor near technician after doxorubicin administration	ND	ND
	Floor between examination tables	ND	ND
	Chemotherapy waste disposal lid after doxorubicin	ND	ND
Room D161	Telephone in cubicle near hallway door (estimated area)	ND	ND
Reception Area	Discharge medical records bin	ND	ND
	Countertop in area behind reception desk	ND	ND
	Reception area floor	ND	ND
	Reception desk near computer	ND	ND
Women's Locker Room	Changing area floor	ND	ND
	Floor near door	ND	ND
Radiology Room (A135)	Room #4 on exam table under X-ray	ND	ND
	Floor next to exam table	ND	ND
	Sandbag used to position animals	ND	ND
Laundry	Floor in front of washer	ND	ND
	Washer loading door (estimated area)	ND	ND

Table. Chemotherapy drugs in surface wipe samples collected on September 13–15, 2010 (continued)

Location	Sample Description	Results, ng/100 cm²	
		Cyclophosphamide	Ifosfamide
Oncology Hallway	Floor directly outside pharmacy mixing room D157	ND	ND
	Floor directly outside the chemotherapy administration room	ND	ND
	Floor directly outside the technician offices	ND	ND
	Floor inside technician office area	ND	ND
	Floor entering technician office from administration	ND	ND
	Floor at corner of hallway away from reception area	ND	ND
	Floor near door to Room D165	ND	ND
Room D158A	Floor near drain in the run area	ND	ND
Room D161	Technician office, on table by door to administration	ND	ND
	Keyboard on the middle desk	ND	ND
Room D165	Conference room table	ND	ND
Ward 1 (D100)	Floor next to animal treated with vincristine	ND	ND
Room D112A	Floor near chemotherapy treated animal	ND	ND
Ultrasound	Floor near drain	ND	ND
Small Animal	Reception area floor near front door	ND	ND
LOD		5	2
LOQ		17	7.3

ND = not detected (result was below the LOD)
( ) Sample results in parentheses were between the LOD and the LOQ, meaning that they have more uncertainty associated with them.

PPE use, 70% reported "always" wearing double gloves when administering chemotherapy drugs, and 60% reported "always" wearing disposable gowns. Several employees reported concerns about being required to re-use disposable PPE items such as gowns because of cost concerns. Most employees demonstrated a good working knowledge of the proper procedures for the disposal of chemotherapy drugs and administration supplies.

Review of the Biological Safety Cabinet and Other Workplace Observations

The Class 2 BSC was certified annually as recommended by CDC [CDC 2007]. According to veterinary hospital records the BSC met the recommended exhaust flow rate of 100 linear feet per minute with the sash open to the typical operating height. The BSC was equipped with a HEPA filter and recirculated 100% of the exhausted air back into the chemotherapy drug preparation room.

Some veterinary hospital employees voluntarily wore elastomeric half-mask respirators equipped with organic vapor cartridges when they prepared and/or administered chemotherapy drugs. We noted that when chemotherapy drug-treated animals were taken to other areas of the hospital or returned home they were no longer visually identifiable as having recently received chemotherapy drugs. A treated animal can spread unmetabolized chemotherapy drugs through biological fluids such as urine, feces, and vomit [Pellicaan and Teske 1999].

We found cyclophosphamide and ifosfamide in a few surface wipe samples, mainly in and around the BSC in the chemotherapy drug preparation room. Although we did not detect doxorubicin, it is important to note that the samples were frozen for approximately 9 months while an analytical method was developed. NIOSH has conducted stability studies of cyclophosphamide and ifosfamide when collected on surface wipe samples, and no recovery degradation was observed [Burr 2011a]. However, NIOSH chemists have observed in laboratory experiments that doxorubicin degraded after being frozen [Burr 2011b]. Therefore, we cannot exclude the chance that doxorubicin may have been present when the samples were collected.

One limitation to this evaluation is that we collected surface wipe samples over 3 days, and this short time period may not be representative of typical exposures. Levels of chemotherapy drugs on surfaces may vary over time depending on patient load, quantities of drugs, and whether proper work practices are followed. Another limitation is that the surface wipe samples were analyzed only for cyclophosphamide, ifosfamide, and doxorubicin, although the veterinary hospital uses other hazardous drugs [NIOSH 2010]. Because the possibility remains that other hazardous drugs may be present or that exposures could be greater at other times, we consider it prudent to control potential chemotherapy drug exposures to levels as low as reasonably achievable.

The absence of cyclophosphamide, ifosfamide, or doxorubicin in air samples is not unexpected considering these drugs are not volatile at room temperature. However, because doxorubicin can degrade when frozen we cannot exclude the possibility that it may have been present when the air samples were collected [Burr 2011a,b]. In this evaluation we learned that Mustargen, a chemotherapy drug that is more volatile than cyclophosphamide, ifosfamide, or doxorubicin, was prepared in the BSC. A sampling and analytical method does not exist for Mustargen on work surfaces or in the air.

We learned that the veterinary hospital was transitioning to preparing Mustargen in a chemical fume hood (which does not recirculate exhaust air) instead of the BSC. We agree that Mustargen should not be handled in the BSC if some or all of the exhausted air is recirculated. Because a HEPA filter does not capture and remove drug vapors, the potential for recirculation exists. However, chemotherapy drugs should not

DISCUSSION (CONTINUED)

be prepared in a chemical fume hood because the sterility of the drug(s) may be compromised.

Three employees reported acute symptoms that they associated with their work. We are unable to determine if the symptoms of headache, nausea, facial flushing, and abnormal menstruation were related to work; however, these symptoms have been associated with occupational exposure to chemotherapy drugs in other studies [Shortridge et al.1995; Connor and McDiamond 2006]. Most employees reported dissatisfaction with their work area's health and safety program, including the lack of written policies on PPE use. Although most interviewed employees reported proper PPE use when administrating chemotherapy drugs, appropriate PPE should be worn at all times during drug administration.

CONCLUSIONS

Cyclophosphamide and ifosfamide, but not doxorubicin, were detected on some surface wipe samples, primarily in and around the BSC. We did not detect these chemotherapy drugs in the air. Because doxorubicin degrades after being frozen [Burr 2011b], we cannot exclude the possibility that this drug may have been present when the surface or air samples were collected. A more volatile chemotherapy drug such as Mustargen has the potential to enter the work area if it is prepared in the BSC because some of the exhausted air is recirculated. We could not determine if the acute health symptoms reported by employees were work related. Recommendations are provided below to limit chemotherapy drug exposure, address employee concerns about their workplace health and safety program, and maintain consistent work practices and PPE use.

On the basis of our findings we recommend the actions listed below to create a more healthful workplace. We encourage the veterinary hospital to use a labor-management health and safety committee or working group to discuss the recommendations in this report and develop an action plan. Those involved in the work can best set priorities and assess the feasibility of our recommendations for the specific situation at the veterinary hospital. Our recommendations are based on the hierarchy of controls approach discussed in Appendix B: Occupational Exposure Limits and Health Effects. This approach groups actions by their likely effectiveness in reducing or removing hazards. In most cases, the preferred approach is to eliminate hazardous materials or processes and install engineering controls to reduce exposure or shield employees. Until such controls are in place, or if they are not effective or feasible, administrative measures and/or PPE may be needed.

Engineering Controls

Engineering controls reduce exposures to employees by removing the hazard from the process or placing a barrier between the hazard and the employee. Engineering controls are very effective at protecting employees without placing primary responsibility of implementation on the employee.

1. Exhaust 100% of the HEPA-filtered air from the BSC to the outdoors [NIOSH 2004].

Administrative Controls

Administrative controls are management-dictated work practices and policies to reduce or prevent exposures to workplace hazards. The effectiveness of administrative changes in work practices for controlling workplace hazards is dependent on management commitment and employee acceptance. Regular monitoring and reinforcement are necessary to ensure that control policies and procedures are not circumvented in the name of convenience or production.

1. Limit access to the pharmacy, chemotherapy drug preparation room, and administration area to required personnel.

RECOMMENDATIONS (CONTINUED)

2. Do not prepare a volatile chemotherapy drug such as Mustargen in the veterinary hospital BSC if any of the exhaust air is recirculated.

3. Consult with university health and safety officials to identify a BSC that does not recirculate exhaust air. This BSC could be used to prepare more volatile chemotherapy drugs until engineering changes are made to the BSC in the veterinary hospital so that 100% of the exhaust air is directed outdoors.

4. Post "Chemotherapy Drug Administration in Progress" signs when preparing and administering chemotherapy drugs.

5. Prohibit food and drink for human consumption in areas where chemotherapy drugs are handled or stored.

6. Keep doors that lead to the chemotherapy drug preparation room and administration area closed. Using self-closing doors may facilitate compliance.

7. Use dedicated cleaning supplies for the chemotherapy drug preparation room and administration area. If possible, store this equipment in the same area where it is used.

8. Improve communication with critical care and nursing care unit, caretaking, and laundry employees about standard operating procedures concerning vomit, urine, and feces from animals that have been given chemotherapy drugs.

9. Either dispose of or properly handle soiled bedding and blankets from animals who have received chemotherapy according to existing veterinary hospital standard operating procedures.

10. Post warning signs outside of the veterinary hospital's comparative oncology building regarding the potential for chemotherapy drug-contaminated animal waste. Staff should use this area of the building for all chemotherapy drug-treated animals.

11. Instruct all employees and students not to place unnecessary items, such as client records, on potentially contaminated examination and chemotherapy administration tables.

12. Identify animals that have received chemotherapy with brightly colored disposable collars or bands to alert staff that vomit, urine, and feces may contain chemotherapy drugs and that these potentially contaminated areas should be cleaned according to standard operating procedures.

13. Create an interdisciplinary group consisting of managers, technicians, interns, residents, and university health and safety department representatives to address the safety and health of personnel who may come in contact with chemotherapy drugs. This committee should meet routinely, communicate with staff, and work cooperatively with the teaching hospital safety committee.

14. Encourage participation in the voluntary, university-administered surveillance program for employees who work with chemotherapy drugs. Additional information on a medical surveillance program is provided in the references [OSHA 1999; NIOSH 2004].

15. Instruct employees and students about safe work practices involving chemotherapy drugs.

16. Involve employees in selecting training topics and in developing training materials.

Personal Protective Equipment

PPE is the least effective means for controlling employee exposures. Proper use of PPE requires a comprehensive program, and calls for a high level of employee involvement and commitment to be effective. The use of PPE requires the choice of the appropriate equipment to reduce the hazard and the development of supporting programs such as training, change-out schedules, and medical assessment if needed. PPE should not be relied upon as the sole method for limiting employee exposures. Rather, PPE should be used until engineering and administrative controls can be demonstrated to be effective in limiting exposures to acceptable levels.

1. Follow the OSHA respiratory protection standard [29 CFR 1910.134] regarding voluntary use of respirators, including providing Appendix D of the OSHA respiratory protection standard [29 CFR 1910.134] to employees.

2. Instruct employees to wear double chemotherapy protective gloves and a protective gown when decontaminating the BSC and when administering chemotherapy drugs [NIOSH 2009]. Because of the risk for latex sensitivity, non-latex chemotherapy gloves are recommended. Manufacturer recommendations concerning the use of disposable PPE should be followed.

References

Burr G [2011a]. E-mail on October 7, 2011, between G. Burr, Division of Surveillance, Hazard Evaluations and Field Studies and J. Pretty, Division of Applied Research and Technology, National Institute for Occupational Safety and Health, Centers for Disease Control and Prevention, U.S. Department of Health and Human Services.

Burr G [2011b]. Telephone conversation on September 29, 2011, between G. Burr, Division of Surveillance, Hazard Evaluations and Field Studies and J. Pretty, Division of Applied Research and Technology, National Institute for Occupational Safety and Health, Centers for Disease Control and Prevention, U.S. Department of Health and Human Services.

CDC [2007]. Primary containment for biohazards: selection, installation and use of biological safety cabinets. 3rd ed. [http://www.cdc.gov/biosafety/publications/bmbl5/BMBL5_appendixA.pdf]. Date accessed: March 2012.

CFR. Code of Federal Regulations. Washington, DC: U.S. Government Printing Office, Office of the Federal Register.

Conner T, McDiarmid M [2006]. Preventing occupational exposures to antineoplastic drugs in health care settings. CA Cancer J Clin. 56(6):354–365.

NIOSH [2004]. NIOSH Alert: preventing occupational exposure to antineoplastic and other hazardous drugs in health care settings. Cincinnati, OH: U.S. Department of Health and Human Services, Centers for Disease Control and Prevention, National Institute for Occupational Safety and Health, DHHS (NIOSH) Publication No. 2004-165.

NIOSH [2009] Personal protective equipment for health care workers who work with hazardous drugs. Cincinnati, OH: U.S. Department of Health and Human Services, Centers for Disease Control and Prevention, National Institute for Occupational Safety and Health, DHHS (NIOSH) Publication No. 2009-106.

NIOSH [2010]. NIOSH list of antineoplastic and other hazardous drugs in healthcare settings 2010. Cincinnati, OH: U.S. Department of Health and Human Services, Centers for Disease Control and Prevention, National Institute for Occupational Safety and Health, DHHS (NIOSH) Publication No. 2010-167.

REFERENCES
(CONTINUED)

OSHA [1999]. OSHA technical manual, TED 01-00-015, Sec VI, Chapter II: Controlling occupational exposures to hazardous drugs. [http://www.osha.gov/dts/osta/otm/otm_vi/otm_vi_2.html]. Date accessed: February 2012.

Pellicaan CH, Teske E [1999]. Risks of using cytostatic drugs in veterinary medical practice. Tijdschr Diergeneeskd *124*(7):210–215.

Shortridge K, Lemasters G, Valanis B, Hertzberg V [1995]. Menstrual cycles in nurses handling antineoplastic drugs. Cancer Nurs *18*(6):439–444.

APPENDIX A: METHODS

Each surface wipe sample was collected using two Whatman filters (42-millimeter diameter) moistened with an extraction solvent composed of 50% acetonitrile and 50% methanol. A 10 centimeter × 10 centimeter disposable template was used to outline a 100-square-centimeter sampling area. The sample area was wiped once with the first Whatman filter, then again with the second Whatman filter. A clean pair of chemotherapy drug resistant gloves was worn each time.

For each surface location sampled the two wipe samples were collectively analyzed by liquid chromatography mass spectrometry/mass spectrometry following a sampling method internally developed by Bureau Veritas North America. The surface wipe sample LODs and LOQs for each drug are as follows: cyclophosphamide (LOD = 5 ng/sample, LOQ = 17 ng/sample); ifosfamide (LOD = 2 ng/sample, LOQ = 7.3 ng/sample); and doxorubicin (LOD = 7 ng/sample, LOQ = 23 ng/sample). All media and field blanks were below the LOD. Results of a storage stability study with cyclophosphamide and ifosfamide showed no degradation of recovery after 7 to 8 months for surface wipe samples stored frozen [Burr 2011a]. On the basis of these results, we do not expect significant degradation of our field samples with respect to these two drugs. However, NIOSH chemists have observed in laboratory experiments that doxorubicin degraded after being frozen [Burr 2011b].

General area air samples for cyclophosphamide, ifosfamide, and doxorubicin were taken using a Quick Take® 30 high volume sample pump operating at 15 liters per minute and collected on a 37-millimeter diameter polytetrafluorethylene filter contained in a three piece black polypropylene cassette. The sampling filter was supported by a stainless steel pad. The air sample LODs and LOQs for each drug are as follows: cyclophosphamide (LOD = 0.5 ng/sample, LOQ = 1.7 ng/sample); ifosfamide (LOD = 0.5 ng/sample, LOQ = 1.7 ng/sample); and doxorubicin (LOD = 0.8 ng/sample, LOQ = 2.6 ng/sample). The sampling method was internally developed by Bureau Veritas North America; the analytical method was the same as was used for the surface wipe samples.

References

Burr G [2011a]. E-mail on October 7, 2011, between G. Burr, Division of Surveillance, Hazard Evaluations and Field Studies and J. Pretty, Division of Applied Research and Technology, National Institute for Occupational Safety and Health, Centers for Disease Control and Prevention, U.S. Department of Health and Human Services.

Burr G [2011b]. Telephone conversation on September 29, 2011, between G. Burr, Division of Surveillance, Hazard Evaluations and Field Studies and J. Pretty, Division of Applied Research and Technology, National Institute for Occupational Safety and Health, Centers for Disease Control and Prevention, U.S. Department of Health and Human Services.

In evaluating the hazards posed by workplace exposures, NIOSH investigators use both mandatory (legally enforceable) and recommended OELs for chemical, physical, and biological agents as a guide for making recommendations. OELs have been developed by federal agencies and safety and health organizations to prevent the occurrence of adverse health effects from workplace exposures. Generally, OELs suggest levels of exposure that most employees may be exposed to for up to 10 hours per day, 40 hours per week, for a working lifetime, without experiencing adverse health effects. However, not all employees will be protected from adverse health effects even if their exposures are maintained below these levels. A small percentage may experience adverse health effects because of individual susceptibility, a preexisting medical condition, and/or a hypersensitivity (allergy). In addition, some hazardous substances may act in combination with other workplace exposures, the general environment, or with medications or personal habits of the employee to produce adverse health effects even if the occupational exposures are controlled at the level set by the exposure limit. Also, some substances can be absorbed by direct contact with the skin and mucous membranes in addition to being inhaled, which contributes to the individual's overall exposure.

Most OELs are expressed as a TWA exposure. A TWA refers to the average exposure during a normal 8- to 10-hour workday. Some chemical substances and physical agents have recommended STEL or ceiling values where adverse health effects are caused by exposures over a short period. Unless otherwise noted, the STEL is a 15-minute TWA exposure that should not be exceeded at any time during a workday, and the ceiling limit is an exposure that should not be exceeded at any time.

In the United States, OELs have been established by federal agencies, professional organizations, state and local governments, and other entities. Some OELs are legally enforceable limits, while others are recommendations. The U.S. Department of Labor OSHA PELs (29 CFR 1910 [general industry]; 29 CFR 1926 [construction industry]; and 29 CFR 1917 [maritime industry]) are legal limits enforceable in workplaces covered under the Occupational Safety and Health Act of 1970. NIOSH RELs are recommendations based on a critical review of the scientific and technical information available on a given hazard and the adequacy of methods to identify and control the hazard. NIOSH RELs can be found in the NIOSH Pocket Guide to Chemical Hazards [NIOSH 2010]. NIOSH also recommends different types of risk management practices (e.g., engineering controls, safe work practices, employee education/ training, personal protective equipment, and exposure and medical monitoring) to minimize the risk of exposure and adverse health effects from these hazards. Other OELs that are commonly used and cited in the United States include the TLVs recommended by ACGIH, a professional organization, and the WEELs recommended by the American Industrial Hygiene Association, another professional organization. The TLVs and WEELs are developed by committee members of these associations from a review of the published, peer-reviewed literature. They are not consensus standards. ACGIH TLVs are considered voluntary exposure guidelines for use by industrial hygienists and others trained in this discipline "to assist in the control of health hazards" [ACGIH 2011]. WEELs have been established for some chemicals "when no other legal or authoritative limits exist" [AIHA 2011].

Outside the United States, OELs have been established by various agencies and organizations and include both legal and recommended limits. The Institut für Arbeitsschutz der Deutschen Gesetzlichen Unfallversicherung (IFA, Institute for Occupational Safety and Health of the German Social Accident

Insurance) maintains a database of international OELs from European Union member states, Canada (Québec), Japan, Switzerland, and the United States. The database, available at http://www.dguv.de/ifa/en/gestis/limit_values/index.jsp, contains international limits for over 1,500 hazardous substances and is updated periodically.

Employers should understand that not all hazardous chemicals have specific OSHA PELs, and for some agents the legally enforceable and recommended limits may not reflect current health-based information. However, an employer is still required by OSHA to protect its employees from hazards even in the absence of a specific OSHA PEL. OSHA requires an employer to furnish employees a place of employment free from recognized hazards that cause or are likely to cause death or serious physical harm [Occupational Safety and Health Act of 1970 (Public Law 91–596, sec. 5(a)(1))]. Thus, NIOSH investigators encourage employers to make use of other OELs when making risk assessments and risk management decisions to best protect the health of their employees. NIOSH investigators also encourage the use of the traditional hierarchy of controls approach to eliminate or minimize identified workplace hazards. This includes, in order of preference, the use of (1) substitution or elimination of the hazardous agent, (2) engineering controls (e.g , local exhaust ventilation, process enclosure, dilution ventilation), (3) administrative controls (e.g., limiting time of exposure, employee training, work practice changes, medical surveillance), and (4) personal protective equipment (e.g., respiratory protection, gloves, eye protection, hearing protection). Control banding, a qualitative risk assessment and risk management tool, is a complementary approach to protecting employee health that focuses resources on exposure controls by describing how a risk needs to be managed. Information on control banding is available at http://www.cdc.gov/niosh/topics/ctrlbanding/. This approach can be applied in situations where OELs have not been established or can be used to supplement the OELs, when available.

Below we provide the OELs and surface contamination limits for the compounds we measured, as well as a discussion of the potential health effects from exposure to these compounds.

Cyclophosphamide

Although OSHA and NIOSH have not established OELs for cyclophosphamide, it has been categorized as a Group 1 Carcinogen (carcinogenic to humans) by IARC [IARC 1998]. It metabolizes in the body to acrolein, which can cause adverse effects in the bladder.

Cyclophosphamide is a chemotherapy drug used for a wide range of neoplastic diseases such as breast and lung cancer, pediatric malignancies, leukemia, and lymphomas. It can be prescribed as a single drug or in combination with other chemotherapy drugs and can be administered via oral tablets or intravenously.

Cyclophosphamide is normally found in a white powder form for chemical stability and is typically brought into liquid solution by the addition of water and infused with sodium chloride, glucose, or glucose/saline solutions. Once in solution, it is recommended that cyclophosphamide be administered to the patient within 8 hours or stored cold (but not frozen) to prevent degradation. The surface wipe samples collected during this evaluation for cyclophosphamide, (as well as for ifosfamide and doxorubicin) were shipped cold from the field to the NIOSH laboratory. These surface wipe samples were then kept frozen for approximately 7 months pending development of an analytical method. There are currently no OELs for cyclophosphamide. However, because of its carcinogenic nature, exposures to cyclophosphamide should be controlled to the lowest achievable levels.

Ifosfamide

Ifosfamide is a chemotherapy drug that is used for a wide range of neoplastic diseases including ovary, testis, lung, breast, and soft-tissue sarcomas. It can be prescribed as a single drug or in combination with other chemotherapy drugs and can be administered via oral tablets or intravenously. Ifosfamide is normally found in a white powder form for chemical stability and is normally brought into solution by the addition of water and infused with sodium chloride, glucose, or glucose/saline solutions.

Ifosfamide is a not designated as carcinogenic to humans by IARC, OSHA, or NIOSH. It has been reported to be mutagenic in bacterial cells through the Ames test. Ifosfamide metabolizes in the body to acrolein, which can cause adverse effects in the bladder. There are currently no OELs for ifosfamide.

Doxorubicin

Doxorubicin is a chemotherapy drug that is used for neoplastic diseases including leukemia, soft-tissue sarcomas, and solid tumors such as breast and lung cancer. It can be prescribed singly or in combination with other chemotherapy drugs and can be administered via oral tablets or intravenously. It is categorized as a Group 2A Carcinogen [IARC 1987], meaning that there is inadequate evidence to designate it as a human carcinogen.

Chemotherapy Drugs in Healthcare Settings

Occupational exposures to chemotherapy drugs may occur through inhalation, skin contact, skin absorption, ingestion, or injection. Inhalation and skin contact/absorption are the most likely routes of exposure, but unintentional ingestion from hand to mouth contact and unintentional injection through a needlestick or sharps injury are also possible [Duvall and Baumann 1980; Black and Presson 1997; Schreiber et al. 2003].

Protection from chemotherapy drug exposures depends on safety programs established by employers and followed by employees. Factors that affect employee exposures include drug handling circumstances (preparation, administration, or disposal), amount of drug prepared, frequency and duration of drug handling, potential for absorption, use of ventilated cabinets, PPE, and work practices. The chance that an employee will experience adverse effects from chemotherapy drugs increases with the amount and frequency of exposure and the lack of proper work practices [NIOSH 2004].

Surveys have associated workplace exposures to chemotherapy drugs with acute health effects, primarily in nurses. These included hair loss, headaches, acute skin and eye irritation, and/or hypersensitivity [Valanis 1993a; Valanis 1993b]. A review of 14 studies described an association between exposure to chemotherapy drugs and adverse reproductive effects [Harrison 2001]. The major reproductive effects found in these studies were increased fetal loss [Selevan et al. 1985; Stücker et al. 1990], congenital malformations depending on the length of exposure [Hemminki et al. 1985], low birth weight and congenital abnormalities [Peel¬en et al. 1999], and infertility [Valanis et al. 1999].

Several reports have addressed the relationship of cancer occurrence to healthcare employees' exposures to chemotherapy drugs [NIOSH 2004]. A significantly increased risk of leukemia has been reported among oncology nurses identified in the Danish cancer registry for the period 1943–1987 [Skov et al. 1992]. The same group [Skov et al. 1990] found an increased, but not significant, risk of leukemia in physicians employed for at least 6 months in a department where patients were treated with chemotherapy drugs.

References

ACGIH [2011]. 2011 TLVs® and BEIs®: threshold limit values for chemical substances and physical agents and biological exposure indices. Cincinnati, OH: American Conference of Governmental Industrial Hygienists.

AIHA [2011]. AIHA 2011 Emergency response planning guidelines (ERPG) & workplace environmental exposure levels (WEEL) handbook. Fairfax, VA: American Industrial Hygiene Association.

Black LA, Presson AC [1997]. Hazardous drugs. Occup Med: State of the Art Rev 12(4):669–685.

CFR. Code of Federal Regulations. Washington, DC: U.S. Government Printing Office, Office of the Federal Register.

Duvall E, Baumann B [1980]. An unusual accident during the administration of che-motherapy. Cancer Nurs 3(4):305–306.

Harrison BR [2001]. Risks of handling cy¬totoxic drugs. In: Perry MC ed. The chemo¬therapy source book. 3rd ed. Philadelphia, PA: Lippincott, Williams and Wilkins, pp. 566–582.

Hemminki K, Kyyrönen P, Lindbohm M-L [1985]. Spontaneous abortions and malfor-mations in the offspring of nurses exposed to anesthetic gases, cytostatic drugs, and other potential hazards in hospitals, based on registered information of outcome. J Epi¬demiol Commun Health 39:141–147.

IARC [1987]. Overall Evaluations of Carcinogenicity: An Updating of IARC Monographs Volumes 1 to 42. Lyon: IARC monographs on the evaluation of carcinogenic risks to humans, Supplement 7. International Agency for Research on Cancer.

IARC [1998]. Some antineoplastic and immunosuppressive agents. Lyon: IARC monographs on the evaluation of carcinogenic risks to humans; vol 26. International Agency for Research on Cancer.

NIOSH [2004]. NIOSH Alert: preventing occupational exposure to antineoplastic and other hazardous drugs in health care settings. Cincinnati, OH: U.S. Department of Health and Human Services, Centers for Disease Control and Prevention, National Institute for Occupational Safety and Health, DHHS (NIOSH) Publication No. 2004-165.

NIOSH [2010]. NIOSH pocket guide to chemical hazards. Cincinnati, OH: U.S. Department of Health and Human Services, Centers for Disease Control and Prevention, National Institute for Occupational Safety and Health, DHHS (NIOSH) Publication No. 2010-168c. [http://www.cdc.gov/niosh/npg/]. Date accessed: January 2012.

Peelen S, Roeleveld N, Heederik D, Krom¬bout H, de Kort W [1999]. Toxic effects on reproduction in hospital personnel (in Dutch). Netherlands: Elsevier.

Schreiber C, Radon K, Pethran A, Schierl R, Hauff K, Grimm C-H, Boos K-S, Nowak D. [2003]. Uptake of antineoplastic agents in pharmacy personnel. Part 2: study of work-related risk factors. Int Arch Occup Environ Health 76(1):11–16.

Selevan SG, Lindbohm M-L, Hornung RW, Hemminki K [1985]. A study of occupa¬tional exposure to antineoplastic drugs and fetal loss in nurses. N Engl J Med 313(19):1173–1178.

Skov T, Lynge E, Maarup B, Olsen J, Rørth M, Winthereik H [1990]. Risk for physicians handling antineoplastic drugs [letter to the editor]. Lancet 336(8728):1446.

Skov T, Maarup B, Olsen J, Rørth M, Winthereik H, Lynge E [1992]. Leukaemia and reproductive outcome among nurses handling antineoplastic drugs. Br J Ind Med 49(12):855–861.

Stücker I, Caillard J-F, Collin R, Gout M, Poyen D, Hémon D [1990]. Risk of spon¬taneous abortion among nurses handling antineoplastic drugs. Scand J Work Environ Health 16(2):102–107.

Valanis BG, Vollmer WM, Labuhn KT, Glass AG [1993a]. Acute symptoms associated with antineoplastic drug handling among nurses. Cancer Nurs 16(4):288–295.

Valanis BG, Vollmer WM, Labuhn KT, Glass AG [1993b]. Association of antineoplastic drug handling with acute adverse effects in pharmacy personnel. Am J Hosp Pharm 50(3):455–462.

Valanis B, Vollmer WM, Steele P [1999]. Occupational exposure to antineoplastic agents: self-reported miscarriages and stillbirths among nurses and pharmacists. J Occup Environ Med 41(8):632–638.

This page left intentionally blank.

This page left intentionally blank.

Acknowledgments and Availability of Report

The Hazard Evaluations and Technical Assistance Branch (HETAB) of the National Institute for Occupational Safety and Health (NIOSH) conducts field investigations of possible health hazards in the workplace. These investigations are conducted under the authority of Section 20(a)(6) of the Occupational Safety and Health Act of 1970, 29 U.S.C. 669(a)(6) which authorizes the Secretary of Health and Human Services, following a written request from any employer or authorized representative of employees, to determine whether any substance normally found in the place of employment has potentially toxic effects in such concentrations as used or found. HETAB also provides, upon request, technical and consultative assistance to federal, state, and local agencies; labor; industry; and other groups or individuals to control occupational health hazards and to prevent related trauma and disease.

Mention of any company or product does not constitute endorsement by NIOSH. In addition, citations to websites external to NIOSH do not constitute NIOSH endorsement of the sponsoring organizations or their programs or products. Furthermore, NIOSH is not responsible for the content of these websites. All Web addresses referenced in this document were accessible as of the publication date.

This report was prepared by James Couch and John Gibbins of HETAB, Division of Surveillance, Hazard Evaluations and Field Studies and by Thomas Connor of the NIOSH Division of Applied Research and Technology (DART). Industrial hygiene equipment and logistical support was provided by Donald Booher and Karl Feldmann of HETAB. Analytical support was provided by Jack Pretty of DART and Bureau Veritas North America. Health communication assistance was provided by Stefanie Evans. Editorial assistance was provided by Ellen Galloway. Desktop publishing was performed by Greg Hartle.

Copies of this report have been sent to employee and management representatives at the facility, the state health department, and the Occupational Safety and Health Administration Regional Office. This report is not copyrighted and may be freely reproduced. The report may be viewed and printed at http://www.cdc.gov/niosh/hhe/. Copies may be purchased from the National Technical Information Service at 5825 Port Royal Road, Springfield, Virginia 22161.

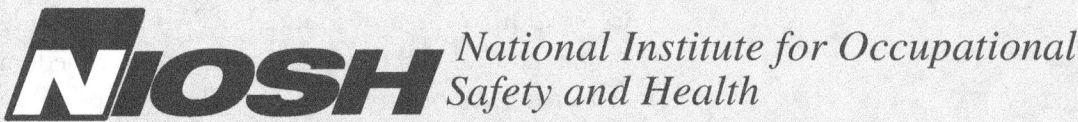

National Institute for Occupational Safety and Health

Delivering on the Nation's promise: Safety and health at work for all people through research and prevention.

To receive NIOSH documents or information about occupational safety and health topics, contact NIOSH at:

1-800-CDC-INFO (1-800-232-4636)

TTY: 1-888-232-6348

E-mail: cdcinfo@cdc.gov

or visit the NIOSH web site at: **www.cdc.gov/niosh.**

For a monthly update on news at NIOSH, subscribe to NIOSH eNews by visiting **www.cdc.gov/niosh/eNews.**

SAFER • HEALTHIER • PEOPLE™

www.ingramcontent.com/pod-product-compliance
Lightning Source LLC
Chambersburg PA
CBHW080936290526

45795CB00007BA/2779